Serious Anti-Aging Skincare Solutions

A Comprehensive Bible with Effective Age Defying Treatments and Natural Remedies for Men and Women Wellbeing

Dr. Jude Nathan

Copyright

Contents

Introduction

In "*Serious Anti-Aging Skincare Solution*," renowned skincare expert we took time to reader on an informative journey to restore youthful, glowing skin. This book contains practical information and insider ideas for severe and anti-aging skin damage. Beginning with a thorough understanding of anti-aging and skincare, we also provide step-by-step instructions for picking the best anti-aging cosmetic surgery and skin care products for various skin types. Readers will discover unexpected facts about oily skin and learn how to choose the best skin care products.

The first step towards minimizing wrinkles is detailed, as are advanced procedures for improving skin appearance and exfoliating to reduce wrinkles. This book discusses essential aspects of selecting a good doctor and care for sensitive skin. It also delves into numerous anti-aging skincare routines and investigates the effectiveness of herbal skincare approaches, providing remedies to the most common skin issues.

The book also includes critical cosmetics tips you didn't know and ten essential skin care suggestions everyone should know. Vitamin C is a powerful anti-agent, and effective wrinkle-reduction methods, including dietary adjustments and simple home treatments, are investigated.

For individuals choosing more intensive procedures, we outlined how facelifts can reduce wrinkles and the general anti-aging benefits of cosmetic surgery. Anti-aging exercises, the role of sleep in aging, and practical suggestions for falling asleep faster are all explored in detail.

With thorough considerations for anti-aging cosmetic surgery, "Serious Anti-

Aging Skincare Solution" provides readers with all the information they need to make informed decisions and attain ageless, radiant skin. This book is an invaluable resource for anyone looking to combat the effects of aging and embrace their most beautiful self.

Description

Welcome to the world of timeless beauty with Serious Anti-Aging Skincare Solution. This book is your best resource for achieving and maintaining youthful, glowing skin. Aging is normal, but you can still look and feel good at any age. This book is intended to equip you with the knowledge, skills, and practices needed to combat the indications of aging effectively and naturally. In this book, you will learn the secret to timeless beauty. Imagine looking in the mirror and seeing a younger, more radiant version of yourself. The Serious Anti-Aging Skincare Solution Book is here to make your dream a reality. This comprehensive book reveals deep secrets and digs into all aspects of anti-aging skincare, providing expert guidance and practical ideas to help you transform your beauty regimen.

This book covers important and relevant topics, including:

Understanding the Science of Ageing:

Before discussing practical tips and treatments, grasping the science of aging and skincare is essential.

What causes our skin to age? How can we slow down the process?

This chapter will reveal the mysteries of aging, giving you a firm foundation of information to help you make informed decisions regarding your skincare practice.

Embracing Natural Skin Care:

Natural skincare stands out as a light of hope in a world dominated by synthetic goods. Learn how natural skincare can help your skin in ways that commercial products frequently cannot. Discover the benefits of herbal skincare and how to include them in your everyday regimen for long-term results.

Making Informed Choices:

Choosing the appropriate skincare products and professionals can be challenging. This book will help you choose the best skincare products based on your skin type and demands. It will also provide valuable insights into selecting the best anti-aging cosmetic doctors and understanding the factors to consider while undergoing anti-aging cosmetic surgery.

Practical Steps to Achieving Youthful Skin:

This book covers everything from the first step to minimizing wrinkles and improving your skin's appearance. Learn how to exfoliate to reduce wrinkles, care for sensitive skin, and effectively treat the most prevalent skin diseases. Important makeup and skincare suggestions will become your new beauty arsenal.

The Power of Lifestyle Changes:

Beautiful skin is more than just the items you use; it also reflects your lifestyle. Discover how to decrease wrinkles with food, anti-aging workouts, and the value of sleep. Learn how getting enough sleep can help you age less and learn valuable methods for falling asleep faster.

Holistic approach to anti-aging:

Embrace a comprehensive approach to skincare, including Vitamin C as anti-agent skin care, home treatments for wrinkle removal, and an understanding of how cosmetic surgery affects aging. This comprehensive guide provides all the information you need to make the best decisions for your skin. Serious Anti-Aging Skincare Solution is more than a book; it's a transformational path to a more young, radiant self. So, are you ready to discover the secrets of ageless beauty? Let's embark on this amazing trip together. Your journey to youthful, beautiful skin begins today.

Tailored Solutions for Each Skin Type:

One size does not fit all, especially in terms of skincare. The Serious Anti-Aging Skincare Solution Book provides personalized recommendations to help you select the right product for your specific skin type. You'll learn to choose products and treatments that complement your natural beauty, whether you have oily, dry, sensitive, or combination skin.

Expert Advice for Cosmetic Procedures:

We offer detailed advice on cosmetic operations for anyone choosing a more professional approach to anti-aging. Learn how to select the best anti-aging cosmetic surgeons and understand the various choices available. You'll learn about everything from non-invasive treatments to surgical procedures so you can make informed decisions about your skincare routine.

The Role of Diet and Exercise:

Your food and physical exercise significantly impact how your skin ages. Learn how specific foods can minimize wrinkles and how anti-aging exercises help you seem younger. This section also includes practical advice on obtaining enough sleep and why it is essential for maintaining healthy, vibrant skin.

Home Remedies and Natural Treatments:

Explore some excellent home remedies for wrinkle removal and other natural treatments that you can quickly implement into your daily routine. These essential, low-cost methods can produce stunning outcomes without requiring costly items or procedures.

Enhancing Your Daily Routine:

Introducing new behaviors into your daily routine can significantly impact your skin's health and appearance. Learn about the first stages of wrinkle reduction, the importance of exfoliation, and how to improve your skin's overall appearance. If you follow these concrete ideas, you'll notice results quickly.

Preparing for Your Anti-Aging Journey:

Starting your anti-aging journey involves more than just products and treatments; it also necessitates a mental adjustment. Prepare to adopt new habits, try new options, and stick to your skincare goals. This book will guide and assist you every step of the way.

And Lots More…..

Aging is a journey, and Serious Anti-Aging Skincare Solution can help you traverse it confidently and gracefully. This book is committed to helping you attain and keep the youthful, bright skin you deserve. Accept the advice, techniques, and treatments offered in these pages, and watch as your skin transforms, revealing a more vibrant, young you. Are you prepared to take control of your skincare and combat the effects of aging? *"Serious Anti-Aging Skincare Solution"* is here to support you every step of the way. Dive into the richness of knowledge, uncover the secrets of youthful skin, and begin your journey to timeless beauty now. Your ageless metamorphosis awaits!

Chapter 1

Understanding Anti-Aging and Skincare

Anti-aging is the process of delaying, stopping, or correcting the indications of old age in the body, especially in the skin. This might include a range of approaches like using skin care therapies, changing one's lifestyle, and receiving medical treatment. Our body systems go through a natural cycle of wear and tear as we age, which can cause wrinkles, fine lines, age spots, and loss of suppleness in the skin. These alterations are addressed by anti-aging methods, which create more young, radiant skin. Moisturizers, serums, and other skincare products containing chemicals like retinol, vitamin

C, and hyaluronic acid, which can help increase collagen formation and lessen the visibility of wrinkles and fine lines, are some popular anti-aging techniques.

Drinking plenty of water, eating a balanced diet rich in antioxidants, taking regular exercise, stopping smoking and heavy sun exposure, and undertaking cosmetic procedures such as laser therapy or injectable fillers are all possible solutions. While it is impossible to prevent the aging process altogether, anti-aging measures can assist to mitigate its effects and ensure a healthy, more youthful appearance.

Skincare

Skincare is the activity of caring for the skin, the biggest element in the human body. To maintain the skin healthy and looking its best, skincare methods include washing, moisturizing, protecting, and correcting it. Regardless of age or skin type, a strong skincare routine is vital for preserving healthy skin. It can aid in the prevention of a range of skin issues, including acne, dryness, sensitivity, and premature aging. A consistent skincare program can also assist to produce more even skin tone, improve skin texture, and reduce the effects of pores.

Cleansers, toners, moisturizers, serums, masks, and exfoliators are examples of skincare products. Skin type, age, lifestyle, and personal interests can all influence which products and routines work best for each individual. Choosing products and techniques that are appropriate for your skin type and issues, and utilizing them consistently over time, is the key to effective skincare. You can obtain healthier, more radiant skin that looks and feels great with the appropriate skincare routine.

Why Some People Age Faster Than Others

Aging is a natural process that happens in all living species and is impacted by several factors including genetics, lifestyle, and environment. While aging is unavoidable, several variables can contribute to premature aging or cause indications of aging to occur sooner than planned. Among these elements are:

- **UV Radiation Exposure**

Extended exposure to the sun's UV rays can damage skin cells, resulting in premature aging, wrinkles, and age spots. Smoking is a major contributor to accelerated aging because it damages collagen and elastin in the skin, resulting in wrinkles, sagging skin, and a dull complexion.

- **Bad Diet**

A diet high in processed foods, sweets, and unhealthy fats can increase inflammation in the body, hastening the aging process.

- **Sleep deprivation**

Prolonged sleep deprivation can cause a variety of health issues, including hastened aging. Prolonged stress can have a range of harmful impacts on the body, including hastening aging. While we cannot control our genetics, they can influence how rapidly we age and the indications of aging that we experience.

You can help to slow down the aging process and lessen the look of premature aging by making good lifestyle choices such as protecting your skin from UV radiation, quitting smoking, eating a healthy diet, getting enough sleep, and managing stress.

The Importance of Caring for Your Skin

As the saying goes, "Packaging is as important as the gift itself," and this concept extends beyond gift-giving. Your outer self, specifically your skin, is just as important as your inner self. While some people recognize the importance of skincare, many do not fully understand its benefits. Skincare products flood the market and tend to do well, with many individuals associating skin care solely with good looks.

However, healthy and glowing skin provides many more benefits beyond appearance. Firstly, it has a positive effect on your mood, making you feel fresher and more energetic.

This, in turn, increases productivity and helps build confidence. Furthermore, the positive energy radiated from your healthy skin can be contagious and affect those around you, leading to a friendlier environment.

In contrast, neglecting skin care can result in an unattractive and dull appearance that can reduce work efficiency and social interactions. Neglect can also accelerate the aging process. Therefore, skincare should not be ignored. Thankfully, skin care is not a difficult task, as there are numerous products available to suit various skin types, including those for oily, dry, and sensitive skin.

Skin care products can also be categorized by their use, such as moisturizers, cleansers, toners, and exfoliants. Additionally, skin care products can target specific skin problems, such as acne, stretch marks, and anti-aging. Skincare products are not the only way to care for your skin, as basic skin care procedures can be incorporated into daily life.

Proper cleansing and moisturizing, for example, can go a long way in maintaining healthy skin. Skincare is not just a superficial endeavor. Healthy skin provides physical and mental benefits, such as increased energy and confidence, and creates a more pleasant and friendly environment.

Neglecting skin care can lead to a dull and unattractive appearance, reduced efficiency, and hindered social interactions. Therefore, taking care of your skin should be a priority, and there are numerous products available to cater to your specific needs.

Chapter 2

What Exactly Is Natural Skin Care

Simply put, 'natural skin care' is skincare that is chemical-free and natural. 'Natural skin care' advocates allowing the skin to care for itself (without the use of synthetic materials/chemicals). Natural skin care is about instilling healthy habits in the way you live your daily life. Many natural skin care methods are the same as those for general body care. So, what are these natural skin care measures? The first and most important natural skin care measure is to drink plenty of water. Every day, 8 cups of water are required. Water aids in the natural removal of toxins from the body. It aids in the overall maintenance of the body and promotes the health of all organ systems (not just the skin). Another low-cost method of natural skin care is general cleanliness. General cleanliness includes taking a daily shower, wearing clean clothes, and lying on a clean mattress/pillow. After all, keeping your skin clean is the key to avoiding skin disorders. The next step is to start exercising regularly. Exercise increases blood flow, which aids in the removal of toxins from the body and keeps you healthy. Exercise also aids in the reduction of stress, which is the biggest threat to good health.

Natural skin care also recommends good food and eating habits. Some foods (for example, oily foods) are associated with triggering acne and should be minimized to the greatest extent possible. Your diet should consist of a diverse range of nutrient-dense foods. Raw fruits and vegetables are known to refresh your body and aid in the removal of toxins. A good night's sleep is also essential to maintain good health and overcoming stress.

A good night's sleep, as a natural skin care measure, delays skin slackening. Another natural skin care therapy is stress reduction. Stress harms the body and health in general. Drinking plenty of water, getting enough sleep, and exercising have all been listed as stress relievers.

Relaxing in a warm bubble bath, listening to music, or participating in your favorite sport are all effective stress relievers. Yoga is yet another stress-relieving technique that is rapidly gaining popularity among the general public. Another natural skin care technique is to avoid excessive sun exposure (by wearing long-sleeved clothing, a hat, and using an umbrella, for example). Sunscreen lotions are ok too.

Many traditional and homemade natural skin care products and measures are also well-known for their efficacy. They are not only natural and simple to implement, but they are also relatively inexpensive. Aside from that, there are numerous natural skin care products on the market.

These include Lavender oil, aloe vera, and others that have no negative side effects.

Chapter 3

Which Skin Care Product Is the Best

There is nothing quite like the perfect skin care product. There is no such thing as 'the best skin care product,' because different people respond differently to various skin care products (based on the skin type to some extent). A brand that is the "best skin care product" for one person may be the worst for another. So, a more logical question would be, "What is the best skin care product for my skin type?" However, this is not entirely logical. We divide people into four categories based on their skin types: dry skin, oily skin, normal skin, and sensitive skin.

This classification, however, is far too broad to be used decisively in choosing the most effective skincare product. Better statements than 'best skin care product' are 'best skin care product for dry skin' or 'best skin care product for oily skin'. But that is exactly what it is - 'better'; it is still inaccurate. So, rephrasing the question to 'What is the best skin care product for me' is the only way to go. Yes, this is the question you should be asking, and unfortunately, there is no simple answer.

Finding the best skin care product for yourself will require some effort on your part. First and foremost, you must comprehend how skin care products function. This is straightforward. All skincare products are made up of two types of ingredients: **active** and **inactive**. The active ingredients are the ones that do the most good for your skin.

The inactive ones simply aid in the delivery of these active ingredients to your skin. For the product to be effective, both ingredients must be beneficial to

your skin (and move on to become the best skin care product for you).
Aside from the ingredients, how you apply your skin care products is critical. This is even more critical. If you do not understand how to apply skin care products, you may spend your entire life looking for the best skin care product for yourself, even if it has already passed you by. Furthermore, the intensity of usage must be determined (of the skin care product). The selection of the best skin care product is also influenced by environmental factors such as temperature, humidity, and pollution level.

How Go Find the Best Skincare Product that Suits Your Skin Type:

- Before applying the best skin care product, wash your skin.

- Instead of plain water, use a makeup remover to remove the makeup before going to bed.

- The potency of active ingredients is limited when used in conjunction with another product, such as a moisturizer. Apply your best skin care product first, followed by a light moisturizer if necessary.

- Use the products on moist, warm skin.

- You will need to try a few different products before you find the best skin care product for you.

- Do not exfoliate excessively or vigorously.

- Adjust your skincare routine per the seasons (winter/summer, for example), changes in environmental factors, and changes in your skin type.

Determining the best skin care product does not happen overnight. Only through experimentation (and awareness) can you discover the "Best skin care product" (for you).

Chapter 4

First Step to Reducing Wrinkles

When it comes to wrinkle reduction, you must take your needs carefully. A variety of variables contribute to the health and well-being of your skin. It is frequently difficult to grasp how products work and why they may fail to work even though they promise to do so. If you're thinking about wrinkle creams and facelifts, you can become broke in the process. Before you do anything else, think about going through a process to find the ideal solution for your needs. The first thing to think about is the condition of your skin. Your skin must be healthy if you want to avoid looking aged too quickly. It will also make you look younger and healthier. Yet, just because you have wrinkles does not imply that your skin is unhealthy. In reality, it simply suggests that you should examine your entire health more closely.

The first step is to improve your diet
Do you eat nutritious meals, such as a diet high in dark-colored vegetables? Do you consume a lot of items that you are aware are unhealthy for you? Do you consume excessively fatty foods? Any of these factors might cause numerous parts of your body to malfunction. If you want to get rid of wrinkles, you need first to improve your general diet.

This entails providing your body with the nutrition it needs through the foods you eat. Many people make the mistake of believing that what they consume is unimportant. If you're gaining wrinkles at a young age, it could be due to a poor diet. Adjust your nutrition to improve your general health and the appearance of your skin.

Enhancing Your Skin Appearance

When it comes to decreasing wrinkles, one of the first things you should do is figure out how to repair the skin on your face and neck. Although some wrinkles are caused by aging, the health of your skin is also vital. In many ways, taking the effort to repair your skin's problems is vital if you want to change the way wrinkles affect your appearance. Improving the quality of your skin now will benefit you in the long run by reducing wrinkles.

One thing you should do is provide your skin with the necessary nutrients. Currently, most of the diets that Americans consume are of poor quality, and even when they are well thought out and carefully planned, they do not provide enough of a punch to improve our health. In many circumstances, adding more nutrients to your diet will be necessary to see meaningful improvement. You should also take a multivitamin. Visit your local health food store, or better yet, look for a trustworthy source online. Buy a high-quality multivitamin.

Those targeted toward providing for older folks may not necessarily be better for you. Consider including a high concentration of vitamins A, C, and E in your diet. These antioxidants are of high quality. Free radicals can be found in your bloodstream. They can be thought of as little particles inhaled. These not only accumulate and trigger life-threatening illnesses, but they also block your cells and make your skin appear sick. Improve your skin's health by providing it with the nutrients it requires to thrive to eliminate wrinkles. The good news is that this doesn't have to be a tough process.

Exfoliating to Reduce Wrinkles

You've probably heard of the chemical peel, which sounds far more terrible than it is. But what if you could obtain the benefits of the chemical peel without leaving your house and decrease the wrinkles on your skin? In reality, there are numerous ways in which this might help you. Start by using a daily regimen of natural and calming cleansers.

Consider including an exfoliating product as well.

When you do this, you increase the overall quality of your skin, giving you a stunning appearance. First and foremost, think about your cleansing approach. Every day and night, you should apply a solution to your face. What you don't want to do is wash your face with hand soap or soap bars.

These creams remove far too many of your skin's natural oils, leaving it dry and even damaged. This skin is unhealthy, it aches, and it is more likely to lead to future wrinkle problems. Buy a high-quality, skin-friendly cleansing program. After that, exfoliate. This is a procedure that just removes the very top layer of skin on your face in a gentle, painless manner. It also aids in the removal of dead skin cells in that area.

This safely stimulates your skin to do something about the need to replace this skin. When fresh skin grows back instead of what was removed, it appears younger and healthier. It's less wrinkled. Washing your face daily is vital for increasing the health of your skin. Make this the time to pamper yourself.

Invest in a high-quality product that can provide you with the assistance you require. Exfoliating is also important.

Keep Away from The Sun

Before you go out and buy an expensive wrinkle cream, take a look at how you're treating your skin. No matter what cream you intend to use, it will be ineffective if you do not properly take care of your skin. Many people make the mistake of using wrinkle cream as a bandage, but that bandage will not work if the cause is not treated first. Nevertheless, before you can do so, you must first examine your existing situation. The sun causes wrinkles in many people.

Our bodies are poisoned by the sun's rays. Most of us only think about using sunscreen when we're going to the beach or when the summer weather is in full swing. The issue is that UV rays penetrate even on gloomy days or in the dead of winter, causing damage to your skin. The more exposed you are, the more likely it is that you will need to repair it.

UV rays are not just the major cause of skin cancer, but they are also a cause of wrinkles. So, what are you going to do? Search for make-up that contains UV protection.

Alternatively, apply sunscreen to your skin before you apply anything else. Make sure you do the same for your children as you leave the house each day. The truth is that sunscreen is necessary if you want to look your age or younger. If you don't use it or don't apply it frequently enough, you incur the danger of UV damage, which includes wrinkles. Don't let these circumstances harm your skin. Sunscreen can help prevent wrinkles from forming.

Other Steps to Reduce Wrinkle

After you've taken the time to improve your body's overall health and well-being, the next step is to improve the quality of your skin in different ways. There are different options available that can significantly or marginally assist you improve your skin and decrease wrinkles.

Each of these approaches has proven to be effective for some people, but there is no assurance that any regimen will work for you. The best way to know your potential benefit is to consult with your dermatologist and cosmetic surgeon.

Here are some options:
- Wrinkle Creams

They are widely accessible and may be beneficial to you. Look for ones that contain Retinal to ensure you receive one that is beneficial. They should say this, or they should indicate they contain Vitamins A, C, and E. Items that purport to be miracle cures are unlikely to be useful.

- Botox

One of the most heavily marketed products now for reducing wrinkles on the face is Botox. If you're looking for a minimally intrusive option, this is the one for you. But, keep in mind that you may need to get it redone frequently. It is a simple choice that may be completed during your lunch break.

- Face Lift

A facelift is a considerably more extreme procedure, but it is not required. Several minor modifications may be made to help increase the skin's capacity to appear fantastic. To erase wrinkles from your skin, both small and significant modifications can be made. These are just a few of the different treatments available to you to help you improve your skin. Take the time to find the one that best meets your needs and falls within your budget.

Chapter 5

How to Choose the Right Anti-Aging Cosmetic Surgeons

When it comes to anti-aging, there are several important factors to consider. It all starts with determining whether cosmetic surgery is right for you. If this is the case, and it is for many people, it is critical to take your time and find the right doctor for the procedure. If you do not invest some time in this process, you may end up needing multiple surgeries when only one would have sufficed. Cosmetic surgeons only get better with practice. They are more confident and precise as they gain experience. When it comes to your cosmetic needs for anti-aging solutions, there are certain things you want to experience.

Finding the Right Doctor

Do your homework properly at home before visiting the doctor's office. The first step is to research the doctor's background. You can do this by looking them up online, using the Better Business Bureau, contacting your local regulatory services, or simply searching for reviews of the person. Other patients who have worked with him, as well as others who have a personal history with other aspects of that doctor, are almost certain to be found. The goal is to determine whether he or she has relevant experience for your requirements.

Next, schedule a consultation with the doctor to discuss your cosmetic surgery options. Follow your interests here. Don't use them if you don't like them, can't understand what they're saying to you, or find that they're not meeting your needs by addressing what's important to you. Most consultations consist of a question and answer session, allowing you to select the person who appears to be the most credible to you. This is also a good time to ask questions about the past and see before and after photos that they've taken themselves.

Will they let you talk to other patients? Do they provide clear answers to your questions? The bottom line is whether or not you like and trust the doctor. If you do, continue. Obtaining additional information and researching your doctor is an important factor. It will make you feel better about the person in whose hands you are entrusting your life. With extra minutes spent doing these things, you will undoubtedly feel better about the entire process and feel better.

Be Careful About Choosing Your Anti-Aging Technique

Did you know that the market for anti-aging products will exceed $42 billion this year? The problem with such a large market is that there are often products and needs that simply do not fit in with those that do. Individuals and businesses are more likely than ever to increase their products in response to rising customer demand, allowing them to share in the profits.

However, many of their products are not worth the price you will pay for them. In this regard, you must pay attention and complete your homework.

Why Does It Matter?

At any given time, there are thousands of products on the market claiming to be the next big thing in anti-aging. Some people believe that certain aspects require their attention more than others. When it comes to anti-aging products, you must exercise caution. Here are some pointers to help you make informed decisions about the anti-aging products you buy and use.

- Do your research

Look up the company that manufactures the product. This can be done directly on the Better Business Bureau's website. Find out what kinds of issues they have, if any, so you don't make the same mistakes as others.

- **Look for feedback from other users**

You can often find reviews of products that will truly meet your needs. Examine the various product categories and then look for product reviews. Find out what other people have discovered about those products. Are they truly worth the price?

- **Discover why they work**

Just because something contains natural elements does not imply that it will provide you with fewer wrinkles. Find out if the science behind it makes sense. A product that cannot provide this for you should be avoided. There is no doubt that you should take the time to find the best anti-aging products for your needs. In many cases, taking the extra time will pay off because you will have the best products and overall investment possible.

Chapter 6

How to Care for Sensitive Skin

Sensitive skin care' is controlled by a few fundamental principles. Nevertheless, before we get into the criteria for sensitive skin care, it's vital to define sensitive skin. Sensitive skin cannot withstand any unfavorable conditions (environmental or otherwise) and becomes easily irritated when in touch with foreign materials (including skin care products). As a result, several products are classified as sensitive skin care products. Yet, the level of sensitivity varies from person to person (and depending on that, the sensitive skin care procedures vary too). Detergents and other chemical-based products often irritate all skin types.

Nonetheless, the damage generally begins beyond a predetermined threshold (or tolerance level). This tolerance threshold is quite low for sensitive skin types, resulting in skin that is easily and quickly harmed.

Some Sensitive Skin Care Tips:
* Only use sensitive skin care products (i.e. the products that are marked for sensitive skin care only). Additionally, examine the product's instructions/notes to determine if there are any unique restrictions/warnings related to the product).

* Even among sensitive skin care products, choose one with the fewest preservatives, colorings, and other substances.

* Avoid using toners. The majority of them include alcohol and are not suitable for those with sensitive skin.

* When conducting laundry or another chemical-based cleaning, wear protective gloves. If you are allergic to

rubber, wear cotton gloves underneath the rubber ones.

* Another important sensitive skin suggestion is to avoid excessive sun exposure. Before going outside in the sun, use sunscreen lotion.

* Avoiding dust and other contaminants is also essential for sensitive skin care. So, before you go out, make sure you're sufficiently covered.

* Utilize soap-free and alcohol-free cleaning products. After you get home from spending time outside, wash your face.

* Do not scrape or exfoliate too vigorously. It can result in redness and even inflammation.

* Do not wear makeup for an extended time. Make use of hypoallergenic makeup removers. As a result, sensitive skin care differs greatly from regular skin care.

Are Cosmetics Useful or Harmful to the Skin?

Having beautiful and healthy skin is something that most people desire. It can boost one's confidence significantly. While some people are naturally blessed with beautiful skin, others may not use any skincare cosmetics due to laziness or fear of skin damage. Despite this, many people still use skin care cosmetics, and the industry is booming. There is a debate on whether skin care cosmetics are useful or harmful. However, everyone desires to look beautiful.

Excess use of skin care cosmetics can be harmful, just as too much of anything is harmful. Therefore, it is essential to find a balance. The first step towards healthy and disease-free skin is to establish and follow a skincare routine. The general recommendation is to cleanse and moisturize daily, and occasionally tone and exfoliate as needed. Additionally, you can use skin care cosmetics as beauty enhancers either as part of your routine or for special occasions.

Choosing the right skin care cosmetic is crucial. Several rules can guide you in selecting suitable products. Firstly, it is essential to use products that match your skin type, whether routine or cosmetic. You can check the label to see whether it is suitable for dry skin, all skin types, or other specific types. It is also important to test the skin care cosmetic before using it by applying it on a small patch of skin, such as the earlobes.

This way, you can check if there is any reaction before applying it to your entire face. Additionally, check the ingredients for chemicals that you are allergic to, and avoid using products that are too harsh on the skin, such as those with high alcohol concentrations. Although they may work in the short term, they may cause lasting damage to your skin. It is also important to use the right quantity of skin care cosmetic products and be gentle when applying them.

Rubbing your skin too hard or trying to squeeze pimples can cause permanent damage to your skin. Finally, if you have any skin disorders such as acne, it is best

to consult a dermatologist before using
any skincare cosmetics.

Chapter 7

Anti-Ageing Skin Care

The concept of "anti-aging skin care" is quite prevalent in today's culture. Many people want to conceal their age using various methods, and some are successful. Anti-aging skin care, on the other hand, is not a miraculous process, but rather a discipline that necessitates a proactive approach. It entails slowing down the aging process and adopting actions to maintain healthy, youthful-looking skin. There are various anti-aging skin care tips available. The first recommendation is to keep up with good eating habits since a well-balanced diet is essential for proper body metabolism. Consuming enough fruits and vegetables, especially raw ones, is vital since they are high in fiber and have a cooling effect on the body. It is also critical to avoid oily and fatty foods, which not only deplete necessary nutrients but also contribute to obesity and other disorders that accelerate aging.

Another key anti-aging skin care advice is to reduce stress. Stress alters the body's metabolism and hastens the aging process. As a result, it is critical to identify appropriate stress management methods, such as sleep, exercise, calming baths, and aromatherapy.

Water consumption is also vital for anti-aging skin care. Water aids in the removal of toxins from the body, keeping it clean and less susceptible to disease. Experts advise drinking 8 glasses of water every day. Daily exercise is an excellent anti-aging skin care treatment. It not only tones muscles but also aids in skin cleansing by emptying away impurities through perspiration. Nonetheless, it is critical to follow an exercise with a warm shower to remove all pollutants.

Another excellent anti-aging skin care measure is to use natural skin care products. Chemical-based cosmetics can be harsh on the skin, so avoid using them excessively. Organic skin care products, whether produced or purchased commercially, are an excellent choice.

Vitamin C-based skin care solutions are a popular anti-aging skin care option. They do, however, oxidize quickly, rendering them hazardous to the skin. As a result, proper storage is essential. If the product turns yellowish-brown, this indicates that the vitamin C has oxidized and it is no longer safe to use.

Finally, protecting the skin from UV rays is critical for anti-aging skin care. Because UV rays have been shown to accelerate the aging process, a decent sunscreen lotion should be part of your anti-aging skincare routine. To summarize, anti-aging skin care is a discipline that necessitates a proactive approach to slow the aging process.

Keeping healthy eating habits, managing stress, drinking lots of water, exercising regularly, utilizing natural skin care products, and protecting the skin from UV radiation are all important measures to achieving youthful-looking skin.

Chapter 8

Herbal Skincare Method

Skin care is not a new notion; in fact, it has been practiced since ancient times. Herbal skin care was possibly the sole way to care for the skin in the past. Yet, synthetic and chemical-based skin care products have mostly replaced traditional herbal remedies. Although herbal skin care recipes were previously widely used, they have since fallen out of favor and are now virtually unknown to a huge segment of the population. This move from herbal to synthetic skin care can be attributed to two major factors. The first reason is that our hectic lifestyles and

laziness make it tough to manufacture natural skin care solutions at home.
The commercialization of skin care is the second cause. Herbal skin care products, too, have become commercialized and must be blended with preservatives to extend their shelf life. As a result, most commercial herbal skin care products are less effective than fresh, handmade solutions. Despite this tendency, there has recently been an increase in interest in natural and herbal skin care practices.

Many people, however, still choose to buy commercial herbal skin care products rather than make their own at home. Aloe Vera is an excellent example of a herbal skin care product that has long been utilized for its natural moisturizing and skin-soothing characteristics.

It can also be used to treat cuts and sunburns. Some herbs having cleansing characteristics, such as dandelion, chamomile, lime blossoms, and rosemary, are summoned when coupled with other herbs, such as tea. Herbal skin care can also benefit from antiseptic

herbs including lavender, marigold, thyme, and fennel.
Toners that are widely used are lavender water and rose water. Tea is another important component in herbal skin care. Tea extracts are frequently used to heal skin damage caused by UV rays. Herbal skin care can also make use of oils derived from botanical extracts, such as tea tree oil, lavender oil, borage oil, and primrose oil.

For increased hydration, fruit oils such as banana, apple, and melon extracts can be added to shower gels. Herbal skin care remedies may include homeopathic treatments and aromatherapies. Herbal skin care is not only good for basic skin care, but it may also be used to treat skin conditions like eczema and psoriasis.

One of the fundamental advantages of herbal skin care is that it usually has no side effects, which is a major reason why many people prefer natural treatments over synthetic ones. Herbal skin care products can also be easily created at home, making them even more tempting. While herbal skin care is unquestionably useful, it is not always essential to forego synthetic skin care products entirely. To address specific skin disorders, some people may need to use clinically established non-herbal products. Remember that everyone's skin is different, and what works for one person may not work for another. Also, the ideal approach to skin care is to discover the right balance of natural and synthetic products for your specific skin type and needs.

Chapter 9

Men's Skincare

The term "men's skin care" may be foreign to some males. Yet, as more men realize the value of skincare, the market for men's skincare products is expanding. While male and female skin is not the same, the concepts of skin care for men and women are very similar. Water-soluble cleansers are suggested as the initial step in any man's skin care program. Cleaning prevents clogged pores by eliminating dirt, grease, and contaminants. Because male skin is naturally oily, cleaning is essential. Cleaning the face should ideally be done once or twice a day, and soap should be avoided. Shaving is an important part of man skin care, and utilizing the right tools and supplies is critical.

Among the most crucial goods to choose from are shaving foam, gel, cream, and aftershave lotion. When choosing shaving products, it is critical to consider the kind of skin, as the degree of oiliness differs from person to person. To limit the danger of cuts, it is advisable to avoid using alcohol-based aftershaves and to use high-quality razors, particularly swivel-head razors. Correct technique is also important, as shaving should be done gently to avoid skin harm.

Because of wider pores and more active sebaceous glands, male skin is often thicker and oilier than female skin. Regular shaving, on the other hand, can easily dehydrate the skin, making moisturizers a crucial element of any man's skincare routine. After shaving, use a moisturizing gel or lotion. Certain shaving foams or gels may even have moisturizing characteristics built in.

Moisturizers should be applied lightly to the face and rubbed in upward strokes. Although men's skin is less susceptible to UV-induced skin cancer, applying sunscreen is still an important element of man's skin care. There are sunscreen moisturizers that also have hydrating characteristics. For individuals looking for a more natural approach to skincare, using male skin care products with natural ingredients such as aloe vera, sea salt, and coconut can be a suitable option.

Men's skin care can also benefit from lavender, tea tree oil, and other naturally antibacterial oils. Taking care of one's skin as a male may appear to be challenging, but it is not as difficult as one might think. A few minutes each day can help ensure good skin now and in the future.

Facts About Oily Skin you didn't Know

To discuss the topic of caring for oily skin, it is necessary to first understand the underlying cause of this skin type. Oily

skin is caused by an overproduction of sebum, a naturally occurring oily substance produced by the skin.
Excess sebum, on the other hand, can cause clogged pores, the accumulation of dead cells, and the formation of acne and pimples, affecting your appearance. As a result, oily skin care is just as important as other skin types' skin care. The primary goal of oily skin care is to remove excess oil from the skin, but it is critical not to completely dehydrate the skin. To accomplish this, it is advised to use a cleanser containing salicylic acid, a beta-hydroxy acid that aids in the slowing of sebum production.

Cleaning should be done twice a day, and more frequently if the weather is hot and humid. Although the majority of oily skin care products are oil-free, it is always a good idea to read the ingredients before purchasing a product, especially if it is labeled as "suitable for all skin types."

Oily skin care is also affected by the degree of oiliness, so some of these "suitable for all" products may be effective for those who are not excessively oily. Only oily skin care products are recommended for people with extremely oily skin.

Following cleansing, an alcohol-based toner can be used as the second step in an oily skin care routine. Excessive toning, on the other hand, can be harmful to the skin. A mild, oil-free, wax-free, and lipid-free moisturizer can be the next step in an oily skin care routine. A clay mask can also be used once a week as an oily skin care measure.

It may be necessary to try a few oily skin care products before determining which one is best for your skin type. If these measures do not produce the desired results, it is recommended that you seek the advice of a dermatologist.

To address the issues associated with oily skin, they may prescribe stronger oily skin care products such as vitamin A creams, retinoids, and sulfur creams.

Chapter 10

Personal Skincare as Daily Routine

Personal skin care is important for maintaining healthy skin. However, the opinion on how to go about it varies from person to person. Some believe that going to a beauty parlor every other day is the solution, while others think that applying some cream or lotion on the skin now and then is enough. Some consider personal skin care an event that happens once a month or once a year, while some people make it a daily routine. The truth is, personal skin care is not complicated, nor is it expensive when you consider the benefits it offers. It simply involves following a routine or procedure that caters to the needs of your skin. Before starting a routine, it is essential to determine your skin type, such as oily, dry, sensitive, or normal, and select the personal skin care products that suit your skin. It may take some experimentation before you find the right products.

Routine for People with Normal Skin

The first step in personal skin care is **cleansing**. A cleanser contains oil, water, and surfactants, which extract dirt and oil from the skin, then water flushes it out, leaving the skin clean. It may take a few trials before finding the best cleanser for you. It is important to use soap-free cleansers and lukewarm water for cleansing since hot and cold water can cause damage to the skin. Over-cleansing should be avoided to prevent damage to the skin.

The second step in personal skin care is **exfoliation**. The skin naturally removes dead cells and replaces them with new skin cells. Exfoliation facilitates this process.

Dead skin cells do not respond to personal skin care products, but they still consume these products, preventing them from reaching the new skin cells. Thus, removing dead skin cells is important for the effectiveness of personal skin care products. Generally, exfoliation takes place after cleansing. You must also understand how much exfoliation your skin needs. Exfoliate 4-5 times per week for oily/normal skin and 1-2 times per week for dry/sensitive skin. In hot and humid weather, exfoliate a couple of times more.

The third step in personal skin care is **moisturization**. This is one of the most important things in personal skin care. Even people with oily skin need moisturizers. Moisturizers not only seal the moisture in your skin cells but also attract moisture from the air whenever needed. However, using too much moisturizer can clog skin pores and harm your skin. The amount of moisturizer your skin needs will become apparent within a week of using it. It is best to apply moisturizer when your skin is still damp. The last step in personal skin care is sunscreen. Many moisturizers come with UV protection, providing double benefits. Such moisturizers are recommended for daily use, regardless of whether it is sunny or cloudy.

Experiment with various personal skin care products and the amount needed to apply to find the recipe that works best for you. However, if you have a skin problem, consult your dermatologist before using any personal skin care products. Personal skin care involves following a routine or procedure that caters to the needs of your skin.

It is important to determine your skin type and select the personal skin care products that suit your skin. A typical routine involves cleansing, exfoliation, moisturization, and sunscreen. It may take some experimentation to find the right products and amount needed to apply. If you have any skin issues, consult your dermatologist before using any personal skin care products.

Chapter 11

Serious Skin Care

Maintaining healthy and glowing skin throughout your life is the essence of 'serious skin care.' As you age, your body's natural skin care mechanisms weaken, which requires responding to the changing needs of your skin. Therefore, 'serious skin care' entails constantly evaluating, analyzing, and changing your skincare routines based on environmental conditions, age, and changes in your skin type. 'Serious skin care' is also about staying informed. With technological advancements and research, new information about skin care emerges every day. Additionally, the composition and nature of skin care products change over time.

Therefore, trying out new products is a crucial aspect of 'serious skin care. 'However, it is advisable to test a new product over a small patch of skin (not facial skin) to observe how your skin reacts to it. Using your skin care products appropriately is also essential to 'serious skin care.'

Applying moisturizers when your skin is damp, using upward strokes to enhance product penetration, removing makeup before going to bed, cleansing before moisturizing or applying makeup, using the correct amount of skin care products, etc., are all good practices that can increase product effectiveness.

Precautions like avoiding contact with detergents and being gentle with your skin are also part of 'serious skin care.' Over-exfoliation, use of low-quality products, and application of strong-chemical-based products can harm your skin. However, some people misunderstand 'serious skin care.' They believe that it involves using large quantities of products as often as possible, which is not true.

Awareness is, therefore, important in helping people understand what 'serious skin care' is truly about. Visiting a dermatologist for treatment of skin disorders is also a vital aspect of 'serious skin care.' Ignoring skin disorders can lead to permanent skin damage.

Therefore, if over-the-counter medication fails to improve the situation, it is essential to seek professional help. Self-surgery, such as squeezing acne/pimples, can result in permanent skin damage and is not recommended.

In summary, 'serious skin care' involves both precautions and preventive measures. It is about being proactive as well as reactive in taking care of your skin. Being proactive about your skin's needs can help reduce the need to be reactive.

Chapter 12

Skin Care Treatment for the Most Common Skin Conditions

Having radiant and healthy skin is an added benefit. Skin care is not just limited to enhancing one's appearance but it also plays a significant role in maintaining good health. Hence, skin care treatment should be taken seriously. In case of a skin problem, proper skin care treatment is necessary. To prevent skin disorders, proactive or preventive skin care treatment should be adopted. Adopting and following basic skin care routines can be referred to as preventive/proactive skin care treatment.

However, despite following this, skin disorders may occur, and preventive skin care only reduces the likelihood of their occurrence. Different skin conditions require different skin care treatments, so let's discuss some common ones. Acne is one of the most widespread issues. The first step in treating acne is to control it and prevent it from getting worse. Wearing tight clothes should be avoided as it can lead to body acne by trapping sweat.

One should avoid touching or rubbing the blemishes since it can worsen the condition. Also, scrubbing or squeezing the blemishes should be avoided. Mild cleansers are recommended for acne skin care treatment, and over-the-counter skin care treatments can be used to treat acne more quickly. Dry skin is generally easy to treat. Moisturizers are the best skin care treatment for dry skin if applied correctly and in the right quantity. It is best to apply moisturizer when the skin is still damp for better results. Overusing or underusing moisturizer should be avoided.

In rare cases where no improvement is seen after 3-4 weeks, it may be necessary to consult a dermatologist for dry skin treatment. Brown spots caused by overexposure to UV rays on sun-exposed skin areas such as the face and hands are a common problem. Sunscreen lotion with high SPF (sun protection factor) such as 15 is an effective skin care treatment for brown spots. It should be used regardless of the weather, and covering exposed skin areas with clothing is another skin care treatment option. If general skin care treatment or over-the-counter medication is ineffective, immediately seek professional skin care treatment from a dermatologist.

The doctor should be informed about any skin care treatments used to date. Thus, the latest skin care treatment (and products) information should be brought along. The dermatologist will recommend a skin care treatment based on the skin condition and the details of the previous skin care treatment such as oral antibiotics, chemical peels, retinoids, etc. which will help in the recovery process.

Chapter 13

Important Makeup Tips You Didn't Know

Makeup and skin care' are generally thought to be the function of women. 'Make-up and skin care' are rarely indulged in by men. Many men take care of their skin, but most men are unfamiliar with make-up. It would be illogical to treat make-up and skin care as separate topics; after all, make-up will only work if the skin is healthy. So, how do you combine make-up and skincare? Here are some make-up and skin-care tips:

1) Keep skin care in mind at all times, whether you are purchasing makeup or applying it to your skin after purchasing it. So, you're purchasing a make-up and skin care product rather than just a makeup product. Examine the ingredients to see if it contains anything to which you are allergic. Check to see if it contains high concentrations of chemicals that could harm your skin.

2) 'Makeup and skin care' also includes product testing before use. So, test the makeup on a small patch of skin, such as your earlobes, and see how your skin reacts to it.

3) Keep track of the expiry date on your cosmetics and never use them after that date. Some products (for example, vitamin C-based products) spoil much sooner than the expiry date if not properly stored.

4) Cleanliness is an important aspect of make-up and skin care. Sharpen your eyeliners regularly, and keep all of your makeup tools clean at all times. You could schedule a monthly overhaul of

your equipment. Your make-up and skincare routine should include keeping your hair clean at all times as part of cleanliness.

5) Another important aspect of make-up and skincare is nail care. Use high-quality nail polish and keep your nails clean at all times. After you've finished cleaning and polishing your nails, apply cuticle oil to the nail's edges.

5) If you have deep-set eyes, use liquid eyeliner rather than a pencil one. This will keep smudging at the deep edges of your eyelids at bay.

6) If you have a skin disorder, such as acne, avoid wearing heavy or chemical-based makeup. If you are unsure about the makeup products you can use while suffering from acne or another skin disorder, consult your dermatologist.
Never squeeze pimples or acne. Remember that make-up and skincare should not be used at the same time.

7) Use a gentle makeup remover (instead of just washing it away).

8) Another essential makeup and skin care procedure is the golden rule: "Never sleep with your make-up on."

9) When applying deodorant, keep the recommended distance between the nozzle and your skin in mind (as mentioned on the deodorant pack). Makeup and skincare should therefore always go hand in hand. Makeup and skincare should not be treated separately.

10 Important Skin Care Tips You Must Know

Healthy skin is one of the most important components of beauty enhancement. This article on skin care tips is an attempt to provide you with the top ten skin care tips. The list of skin care tips is limited to ten because anything more would not only be difficult to remember but would also overshadow the more important skin care tips.

Let's take a look at the top ten skin care tips:

1) One of the most important skin care tips is to understand your skin type. This is significant because not every skin care product is suitable for everyone. All skin care products specify the type of skin they are intended for.

2) Drink a lot of water,' says the doctor. This will not keep your skin moist, but it will aid in the overall maintenance of your health (and in turn your skin). This may appear awkward to some, but it is an important skin care tip.

3) Cleanse your skin regularly (1-2 times every day). This a very effective skin care tip for removing dirt and other harsh elements from your skin. Cleaning is especially important after leaving the house (and hence exposed to pollutants, dust, etc). This skin care tip also recommends cleansing with Lukewarm water (hot and cold water, both, cause damage to your skin)

4) Be gentle, it's your skin after all. Scrub/exfoliate gently and infrequently. Similarly, don't use too many or too few

skin care products. This is a must-follow skin care tip.

5) Always keep your skin moist. This is an extremely important skin care tip. Don't let your skin dry out. Dryness causes the skin's outer layer to break, resulting in a rough and unappealing appearance.

6) Make use of moisturizers and emollients. Moisturizers are most effective when applied while the skin is still damp.

7) Avoid using soap on your face. Soap should only be used from the neck down. A small but crucial skin care tip.

8) Wear sunscreen to protect yourself from the sun's harmful UV rays. You can use sunscreen-infused moisturizers during the day. Use them even if the sky is cloudy. UV rays are known to cause skin cancer, so follow this skin care tip religiously.

9) Exercising and getting enough sleep are also important not only for skin care

but for overall health. Lack of sleep can cause wrinkles to form beneath your eyes, and a lack of exercise can cause your skin to sag. Furthermore, exercise and sleep aid in stress reduction. So, in addition to being a skin care tip, this is a health care tip.

Handle skin problems with caution. This skin care tip emphasizes the importance of not ignoring any skin problems. Before using a skin care product, consult your dermatologist (lest you do end up harming your skin even more).

10) Get rid of stress. Everyone is aware of the negative effects of stress; however, it is sometimes necessary to state the obvious (and hence this skin care tip found its place here). Yes, stress is bad for your skin. So, take a break, soak in a warm bubble bath, or simply sleep well.

Chapter 14

Vitamin C as an Anti-Agent Skin Care

Vitamin C is frequently regarded as an anti-aging or wrinkle-fighting agent. In scientific terms, the primary goal of 'Vitamin C skin care' is to increase collagen synthesis (a structural protein that is found in the skin). The ability of 'Vitamin C skin care' to combat free radicals, which cause skin damage, is an additional benefit.

Challenges with Vitamin C Skincare

Vitamin C skin care is confronted with significant difficulties today. This is due to the oxidative nature of Vitamin C beauty products. When the Vitamin C in the Vitamin C skin care products comes into contact with an oxidizing agent (e.g., air), it oxidizes, rendering the Vitamin C skin care product completely worthless. The oxidized Vitamin C gives the Vitamin C skin care product a yellowish-brown color. This is something you should look into before purchasing a Vitamin C skin care product. Even after purchasing a Vitamin C skin care product, you must store it properly and ensure that it is still safe to use (i.e. it has not developed a yellowish-brown texture).

The producers of Vitamin C skin care products have attempted to address this (oxidation) issue in several ways (and research on Vitamin C skin care products is at the top of their list). One method for retaining the efficacy of Vitamin C skin care products for an extended time is to maintain a high concentration (say, 10%) of Vitamin C.

This raises the price of Vitamin C skin care products. Vitamin C skin care products are already reasonably priced, and raising the price will put the producers out of business. Another option is to use Vitamin C compounds (like ascorbyl palmitate and magnesium ascorbyl phosphate).

These are not only more stable, but they are also less expensive. Even though derivatives-based products are not as successful as Vitamin C skin care products, their oxidation resistance is a valuable feature that makes them stand out. Furthermore, these are known to be less irritating. When discussing the efficacy of Vitamin C skin care products, bear in mind that not everyone's skin reacts to Vitamin C treatments. So, it is not a magical potion in any way.

If you don't notice a difference in your skin, it could be that your skin isn't responding to treatment. As more research is conducted, we can only keep our hopes high and wait for better findings on the challenges 'Vitamin C skin care' is facing presently.

Chapter 15

Best Ways to Reduce Wrinkles

Many of us look forward to being able to reduce wrinkles. The skin ages in the same way that the body does. The sun, our diets, and even our inherited genes all play a role in how much we have to deal with. But One thing is certain. If you would rather not look your age, wrinkles are something to consider. All of us have been programmed to believe that wrinkles are a sign of aging. However, keep in mind that wrinkles can appear at any time in your life. You may appear to be older than you are. One of the most crucial things you can do to improve the health of your skin is to educate yourself about it. Begin by delving into the definition of a wrinkle. It's a ridge where the skin no longer lies flat. Fine wrinkles appear as tiny lines, but they are the precursors to much more noticeable wrinkles.

Is There a Way to Get Rid of Wrinkles?

Wrinkles are folds of your skin that form for a variety of reasons. In theory, they are caused by the skin becoming more elastic and the tissue beneath the skin becoming too loose or being partially removed. Why did you feel the need to get wrinkles? Wrinkles are a natural part of the aging process for everyone. As a result of the loss of collagen beneath the skin, the skin becomes looser. When this occurs, the skin will naturally fold with gravity.

Some people's excessive wrinkles may be caused by excessive sun exposure, a lack of a healthy diet, or even hereditary factors. Is there anything you can do about these circumstances? There are

some. There are numerous options available to you.
Begin by providing your body with the nutrients it requires to keep your skin looking great.

There are also over-the-counter wrinkle treatments. Some of these are effective, while others are not. To replace the missing collagen, you can use plastic surgery or chemical injections. There are several ways to improve the appearance of your face and skin.

5 Most Effective Ways to Reduce Wrinkles

Most people will want to think about wrinkle reduction at some point. People frequently do not realize they are aging until they look in the mirror for the first time and notice wrinkles. Sure, it took a long time for them to arrive, but that doesn't mean you saw it coming. Furthermore, wrinkles will occur for many people regardless of what they do. It's in your blood! These facts, however, are not always understood. Consider these factors when looking for a solution that will allow you to remove the wrinkles on your face.

1. **Eat the right foods**:
Include dark green vegetables, deep reds, oranges, and other colors in your diet. Consuming these items will provide your body with the nutrients and antioxidants it requires to keep your blood flowing. This aids in keeping your skin hydrated and fighting wrinkles.

2. **Use a sunscreen protector**
Even in the winter or on cloudy days, UV rays penetrate and your skin requires protection. The sun is the leading cause of early wrinkles.

3. **Exfoliate your skin**
If you give your skin a weekly facelift, it will always look young. There are numerous creams and washes available to assist you as well. It can be as simple as using them to wash your face.

4. When shopping for wrinkle creams, look for those that contain Vitamins A, C, and E. These are excellent for fighting

wrinkles and bringing new life to your skin.

5. **Remove makeup and excess oils from your face regularly**:
If you do not provide your skin with the necessary care, you will develop wrinkles. However, avoid drying out your skin. Debris removal from your pores is essential for healthy-looking skin and fewer wrinkles.

Although no product can guarantee that it will remove the wrinkles on your face and neck, there are many ways that you can improve the quality of your skin. If you seek out high-quality products and maintain good health habits, the result will be a more attractive you.

Chapter 16

Reducing Wrinkles Through Diet

Experts agree that most Americans do not understand the importance of eating a healthy diet. However, if you are getting older, this is the major time in your life to consider this factor. What you eat has a significant impact on your healthy glow. If you don't eat well, you're more likely to develop the dreaded wrinkles. One of the most important things you can do to reduce wrinkles is to eat a well-balanced diet. Numerous factors influence your body's health. While bacteria and genetic background do play a role in wrinkles, they are not the only factors. Several women and men will develop wrinkles before the age of thirty. This has a lot to do with the healthy diet you are most likely not getting.

Is There a Diet for Wrinkles?

What effect does your diet have on wrinkles? First and probably most important, understand that wrinkles can be caused by a variety of factors, including the body's inability to retain a substance known as collagen. When your body lacks this, your skin becomes looser, resulting in wrinkles.

You can walk away with fewer wrinkles and better skin care if you give your body the necessary nutrients to power through these situations. More vegetables are one thing to think about eating. Vegetables contain antioxidants, which are true warriors in the fight against a variety of health risks.

These substances enter the bloodstream and clean out the cells. This allows blood to flow more easily through the body.

When this occurs, your skin appears amazing and full. Antioxidants play an important role in wrinkle reduction.

What foods should you consume? Consume an antioxidant-rich diet to prevent the wrinkles you already have or to help stop new ones from appearing. Consume a diet rich in fresh vegetables, lean meats, and unsaturated fats. These actions will result in a healthy diet that will provide significant benefits to your overall health. When you provide your body with the tools it requires, it will be better able to reduce wrinkles and provide you with glowing beautiful skin.

Buying Wrinkle Cream Over the Counter

There are several different over-the-counter cream brands that you could use to reduce wrinkles. Many times, these are advertised as a miracle wrinkle treatment, allowing you to simply apply the cream and see the wrinkles fade away. Do you realize how close to impossible that is? It took more than a few days for your skin to produce those wrinkles, and it will most likely take well over a few days to remove them.

Now, before you dismiss these creams as something that simply does not work, consider how they might work for you.

Some over-the-counter wrinkle creams have shown some advantages in wrinkle reduction, but not all. If you intend to use this method to combat wrinkles, make sure that the product you choose contains the following ingredients, which have been connected to improving skin quality.

While not all of these ingredients have been thoroughly researched to provide full guarantees, they appear to be the most effective in combating wrinkles and restoring a youthful appearance to the face.

• Vitamin A

This antioxidant has been a pioneer in wrinkle reduction. Look for skin creams and wrinkle reducers that contain this, but make sure it is in the highest concentration possible. This vitamin aids in the complete collapse of free radicals, which cause the breakdown of skin cells.

• Hydroxy Acids

Consider this exfoliating product. You want a wrinkle cream that does this because it will take away the top layers of aged skin and assist your skin in producing new, healthy-looking skin.

• Alpha Lipoic Acid

This is an antioxidant that can aid in cell membrane penetration. This helps to eliminate free radicals, which break down the cells in your skin. This also enhances the performance of other antioxidants that perform the same function. Vitamins C and E are excellent choices. If you want to reduce wrinkles with over-the-counter creams, lotions, and agents, look for those that contain a high concentration of these ingredients. They are the most beneficial in terms of improving the appearance of the skin and limiting the appearance of wrinkles.

Do Over-the-Counter Medications Work?

There are thousands of products on the market that promise to offer a variety of wrinkle-reducing elements. If you walk into a department store and look at the product counters, you will almost certainly find an entire section dedicated to wrinkle creams of one kind or another.

Do they have any effect?

If you ask the sales assistant if they do, they will almost certainly tell you about some miraculous product they used.
But, in reality, many factors influence whether or not the product will work. But the bottom line is that not all wrinkle creams work. It is up to you, however, to find those who do work. To assist you, here are a few pointers to help you find the best answer to your wrinkle problems.

1. Look over the ingredients. Take a look at the ingredients before making a purchase, whether online or in person. Sure, there are some words you don't recognize. However, there should be several beneficial vitamins included.

Vitamin A is the most essential because it is one of the most effective wrinkle fighters available. Look for vitamins C and E as well.

2. Have a look around the internet. The Internet has more product possibilities than any store. Furthermore, the name brand is unquestionably

3. There is no obvious sign of the product's quality. It may not work at all for you, whereas another generic will. Keep your options open in this situation.

4. Anticipate what others will say to you. Wrinkle creams are not cheap, so you will need the guidance and professional opinion of others. Make certain that you are only trying to compare their situations to your own if they are identical.

Also, keep in mind that they may or may not have used the product as directed. However, customer reviews of various wrinkle-reducing products will assist you in making a decision. You deserve

quality, which is why you should only use wrinkle creams that can provide it.
The truth is that many can help you, but there are just as many, if not more, who will lead you astray.

Chapter 17

Reducing Wrinkles with Botox

Consider Botox to reduce wrinkles. Several people are searching for a way to get rid of the wrinkles that have crept up on them throughout their lives. Even though most people are unaware that healthy skincare and a healthy diet can minimize the number of wrinkles they have, many are contemplating chemical injections such as Botox. If you're thinking about it, consider these Botox and similar facts first. What Exactly Is Botox? Botox is prescribed via injections into the skin's underlayers. It works by relaxing the facial muscles that engulf your wrinkles.

This makes them less visible. Since the muscles are relaxed, the skin lays smoother, resulting in fewer visible wrinkles. Botulinum toxin type A, a purified and reliable form of the toxin that causes botulism, is the substance that is injected.

The injections are not painful and are frequently thought to be a quick fix for wrinkles. Is this, however, the best option for you? What Can You Do with It? Botox can be used in many different ways and will have the same impact in each. The corners of your eyes, the frown lines that run between your brows and the bridge of your nose, your forehead, and the wrinkle bands in your neck are the most common places for them. What you need to know is that Botox will not work on wrinkles incurred by sun exposure. It also does not treat all wrinkles on your face. Also, for some, the thickness and type of skin you have will influence how potent Botox is for you.

Is Botox the right procedure for you?
Think about talking with a specialist to find out if you meet the criteria and if it

would be effective for your wrinkles. Keep in mind that Botox is not a cure and that you will need to repeat the procedure to keep the wrinkles at bay. As more wrinkles appear, it may become less productive for you. Nonetheless, many women are discovering that Botox is the appropriate solution to their need for wrinkle reduction.

Making Use of Home Remedies

Did you think you could get rid of your wrinkles with some simple home remedies? The truth is that numerous items in your home can help improve your health. Some of these treatment options have been handed down for thousands of years. Why have they survived this long? Perhaps because of how useful they can be. While there is no way to get rid of all of your wrinkles, several of these brands can provide a variety of benefits by preventing wrinkles from escalating and making them less noticeable.

Here are some great home remedies for getting rid of wrinkles.

1. Get a massage
A good massage will not only make your body feel good, but it will also make you look good. A massage will stimulate the flow of blood through your body, allowing it to clean out and restore cells more efficiently and quickly. Your muscles are also looser, which aids in the relaxation of wrinkles.

2. Prepare a solution of turmeric powder and sugarcane juice (one part turmeric powder to one part sugarcane juice) to use on wrinkles. Apply to wrinkled areas daily to see results.

3. Green Thompson seedless grapes can also be effective: Apply the juice to your face after squeezing them. Allow it to sit for about twenty minutes before rinsing.

4. Apply green pineapple juice to your face daily: Allow it to sit for at least ten minutes. This will also aid in the removal of cracked skin.

5. Apply the core of the pineapple to your skin for finer lines: Allow it to sit in the

sink for at least ten minutes before rinsing with warm water.

This will help to remove some of the fine wrinkles that you know will eventually become larger ones. Home remedies for wrinkle reduction are safe unless you are sensitive to the product. There are thousands of other options available.

If you want to discover the most effective home remedies for your skin care needs, look in your pantry and forget about the expensive skin care regimens available.

Using Laser Resurfacing

If you have wrinkles, whether you want to accept them or not, you need to do something about them. You may have fine lines forming under your eyes. Alternatively, you may be looking at laugh lines that are no longer amusing.

Wrinkles are a sure sign that you're getting older. But keep in mind that you are only as young as you feel. With that in mind, take into account how laser resurfacing might be the treatment

you're looking for to lessen the signs of aging that are appearing on your skin.
First and foremost, what exactly is it? Laser resurfacing is exactly as it sounds. Your old, affected, and aged-looking skin is eliminated using a laser. This enables your glands to release new skin that is healthier, younger looking and has fewer visible wrinkles. Nothing, in all effects, can truly fix every wrinkle on your face. However, laser resurfacing has shown to be incredibly useful to a wide range of people.

Laser resurfacing is effective in a variety of situations. It is most effective on fine wrinkles, but it also works on moderate wrinkles. It can also help with other aging symptoms such as liver spots and aging spots. If you have skin that has been damaged by the sun, you can also get help. Did you suffer from acne as a child, leaving you with scars? All of these things could potentially benefit from laser resurfacing.

The procedure is not difficult. A small light energy laser will be used to quickly and effectively destroy the very top layer of skin on the areas to be treated.

It will then heat the underlying skin, known as the dermis, sufficiently to stimulate skin growth. Because the top layer of skin was removed, your body will need to recreate the area with new skin. The skin that comes in will be fresh and have fewer wrinkles.

Is Laser Resurfacing the Best Wrinkle Treatment for You?

Many people have used it with great success. The best solution for you is to find the best-skilled specialist to do the work for you, as skill plays a significant role in the procedure's quality.

Chapter 18

Reducing Wrinkles Through A Facelift

Do you want to understand how to enhance the quality of your skin? Are you trying to figure out how to remove the age lines that life has bestowed upon you? You might then consider a facelift. A facelift is not as drastic as it sounds, but it is still an elective surgery with some complications and adverse outcomes, just like any other surgery. Is this the best option for you? What exactly is Facelift All About? A facelift is a process that can do several things for you. For starters, it will stiffen loose skin on your face and neck. This aids in the removal of existing wrinkles.

A facelift is drastic enough to make even the most prominent wrinkles appear less visible if not completely removed. It is beneficial for the area around the nose and mouth, as well as for extracting fat from the neck area. If you're worried about your body's ability to look young, this is one way to deal with it.

There are several types of facelifts available. The smallest, for example, are called feather lifts, and they require little or no invasive surgery to help eliminate a few wrinkles in the desired location. The deep plane lifts provide more in-depth coverage, helping to tighten large muscle groups in contrast. You may want to consider a transplant if you have a facelift.

These can be positioned in your cheekbones, jaw, or other areas to help establish the natural beauty of your skin and remove wrinkles. There are numerous variations in the costs of a facelift. Many other factors influence that decision. For example, the expertise and reputation of your doctor will influence the cost.

Different parts of the country have different price ranges, with California and New York being the most expensive. Furthermore, the type of procedure performed will determine the extent of the cost.

Is a facelift the best option for you? Many people have undergone this process and walked out of the doctor's office looking 10, 20, or more years younger due to wrinkle reduction.

Chapter 19

Dealing with Anti-Aging

Anti-aging is a popular phrase these days. However, there are numerous ways to achieve better skin, better health, and even defy the odds of aging. Each part of your body appears to function less optimally as you age, which frequently indicates where the issue lies. Can You Defy the Odds with Anti-Aging? However, if you can confidently provide for the needs that your body is now missing, you may be able to find the rewards that you seek while still looking as young as you feel. When you do a simple search for anti-aging options, you will notice a plethora of them. But, before you do that and get inundated with numerous spam emails that seem to provide no actual benefit, consider what your body requires. Often, it is simply a matter of meeting your body's new demands. Your parents gave you the best nutrition possible when you were born so that your body could grow. Later, as a young adult, you discovered how to eat properly and do the things required to maintain your weight. You must consider and provide for your body's new needs as you age. That's the key.

What does your body need that you aren't providing? One of the first things to consider as you age is calcium for strong bones. Without added calcium, your body's need for calcium increases, and calcium must be obtained from your bones.

This weakens bones, causes pain, and can even lead to further injury. But what about anti-aging skin care? The skin ages in its unique manner. The body no longer produces as much collagen as it once did, resulting in wrinkles. Simply put, there isn't enough fat under the skin to support the skin.

Simply invest in a nutritious, antioxidant-rich diet to address this issue. Alternatively, you can consider injections and cosmetic touch-ups to help restore some of that lost collagen. Discovering what your body requires and then supplementing it with additional resources to help meet those requirements is a wonderful way to prevent aging and defy the odds. You can boost your body's ability to resist aging by meeting your needs now, while you still can do so.

Chapter 20

Calorie Restrictions for Anti-Aging

One method of anti-aging technique that appears to be quite effective is limiting the number of calories consumed. By no means is this theory fully understood, but it is something that should be carefully considered. **Why does calorie restriction aid in weight loss?** The evidence is clear, but most doctors are baffled as to why this occurs. Nonetheless, it is an excellent option for people looking for a way to combat aging signs all over their bodies. **What is the most likely scenario**?

Calorie restriction aids in the prevention of disease and the extension of life. The idea behind this type of anti-aging solution is that lowering your calorie intake will reduce the amount of insulin your body produces. With this insulin reduction, the signs of aging will be reduced. This is because insulin accelerates the aging process. We see opportunities from reduced calories because those calories have lower oxidative stress. You've probably heard about the advantages of antioxidants.

By eating foods in a less processed manner, less "bad" enters the body, with the potential for more "good," antioxidants to enter. This, too, can help you improve your overall health. To make calorie restriction work for you, you must first consult with a dietician to learn which foods are essential and which should be avoided. You don't have to eliminate everything, but every calorie must count in this plan, rather than allowing empty calories into your diet.

You should also avoid meal replacement products because they rarely provide the same advantages as good, wholesome nutrition. You can even learn which foods are regarded as superfoods because they can provide high levels of nutrition while being low in calories.

If you decide to use calorie restriction as an anti-aging method, do so with the help and advice of your doctor. You should consider what you eat rather than simply cutting back on how much you eat. The goal here is not to go hungry in any way. It is instead to replace high-calorie, bad foods in your diet with foods that are considered highly healthy and have lower calorie counts.

Chapter 21
Cosmetic Surgery and Anti-Aging Effect

There is no denying that cosmetic surgery is one of the most potent ways for people to get anti-aging help. The term cosmetic refers to something done to improve the appearance of something rather than its function. However, the goal of cosmetic surgery is to improve more than just the appearance of your skin, but also how you feel about yourself. If you believe that your wrinkles are lowering your self-esteem, it may be healthy for the body to invest in some form of cosmetic surgery. **What Has Been Spent**? The cosmetic surgery industry is currently expanding by leaps and bounds. The number of procedures performed grows at an alarming rate each year. These methods will be performed on both men and women. Furthermore, there is no doubt that the cost of doing so will rise from $20 billion in 2003 to well over $50 billion, if not more, by 2007. Cosmetic surgery is most commonly used by people aged 35 to 50. Is this, however, a bad thing?

Is It Harmful?
There can't be anyone who says that cosmetic surgery is always bad unless it puts you at risk for other health issues. However, there are risks associated. You may need more than one operation if you do not have a skilled surgeon. Every year, there are a handful of surgical errors. Furthermore, there is nothing cheap or inexpensive about this anti-aging solution.

However, cosmetic surgery improves self-esteem, which many scientists and medical professionals believe can help an individual improve their overall health.

You can do more physically and mentally if you are positively motivated. When you are depressed, illness and disease become more prevalent. As a result, there are health benefits to cosmetic surgery that will improve the patient's outlook. Is cosmetic surgery appropriate for you? You are the only one who can weigh the costs, risks, and overall benefits. If you choose this path, you will have to invest in research to find the best doctor for your procedure. Risks are reduced and procedures are more effective when they are in the hands of qualified individuals.

Chapter 23

Anti-Aging Exercises to Engage In

Exercise is commonly thought to be beneficial, but when it comes to anti-aging needs, it may be something to keep an eye on. By far, you must incorporate some form of exercise into your daily routine. However, you should not overdo it with exercise. Many people who are starting to show signs of aging should exercise greater caution to this limit. You can effectively control your aging requirements with a few guidelines tools.

Regular Exercise Is Needed

You must exercise regularly.

You use the fuel that you have placed in your body by moving it. You keep it active; you keep that fuel burning so that it doesn't add extra pounds to your abdomen or somewhere on your body. Weight gain can be especially damaging to health, causing a person to age faster than necessary in many cases. Losing weight has the potential to improve your health tenfold. If you can do this, you will see progress.

Too Much of Anything Isn't Good

However, when it comes to any anti-aging needs you may have, you should keep in mind that too much, or excessive, exercise is not good for you. Exorbitant exercise, such as running a marathon every weekend, is thought by many doctors to be harmful to your skin.

The issue here is an excess of cardiovascular aerobic exercise. If you do this type of exercise without providing your body with the necessary antioxidants, you will easily find yourself dealing with irritated skin. Your body has several needs, one of which is the proper amount of antioxidants to remove unwanted toxins and reduce oxidative damage. Exercising at high levels causes more oxidative harm to your complexion as part of the process. Keep in mind that strenuous exercise puts a strain on many parts of the body, which include the skin. Without replacing those needs with increased antioxidant levels (or adding significant amounts of extra antioxidants to your diet), your skin will age more quickly than if you only exercised moderately. While this level of exercise is fine when you offer adequate antioxidant protection, limiting the stress on your body will enhance your aging.

Do Anti-Aging Products Work?

As you walk through the aisles of your favorite department store, you notice a plethora of anti-aging products. They call out to you, promising to make you look better than you have since you were a teenager. Many make unrealistic promises, and unfortunately, many of them will not work for you. However, many can provide exactly what you're looking for: improved skin, healthy-looking skin, and youthful-looking skin. It is possible, and there are some alternatives to consider.

Understanding What Works

The most difficult thing to overcome is determining which products are effective and which are not. Here are some pointers to help you figure out which anti-aging products are the best on the market.
 • Expand your knowledge
Learn why they work. What is their commitment to you? Does it make scientific sense to work this way? Finding out not only what they promise to do but also why they work can often help you eliminate those that don't make sense or aren't right for you.

 • Learn from the experts
Others have most likely used the anti-aging product before you. Take the time necessary to learn about their experiences. Determine whether or not they would recommend them to others. This is simple to do on the Internet.

- Research the company

Companies that consistently put products on the market that provide no benefits to the majority of people are frequently reported to the Better Business Bureau. You can also learn more about the company and its products by visiting the Consumer Reports website. Either of these options will provide you with more information about whether or not this company is genuine in its claims of anti-aging products that work.

Additional Tips

Another common issue that many people who use anti-aging products encounter is that they do not work. However, this is not because the product does not have the potential to work, but because they did not use it correctly. That allows for the worst-case scenario. Following the instructions will undoubtedly improve your body's ability to reap the full benefits of the product. Anti-aging products that have been thoroughly researched and used as directed can provide a great deal of assistance and well-being to an individual. You can benefit from them in terms of improved health and wellness.

Chapter 24

How Getting Enough Sleep Can Reduce Aging Effect

re you getting enough sleep? If you're looking for an anti-aging technique that works for you, make sure you're still getting enough sleep. There is no doubt that your body will age as time passes. However, the amount of aging that you witness in your physical looks and health can be managed to a certain degree. Whatever path you take to improve your overall health and reduce the signs of aging, make sure sleep is part of the plan.

Sleep Is Necessary Sleep is your body's way of healing and repairing itself.

Your body uses your energy and resources while you sleep to boost your immune system, repair cells, grow, and even enhance your health. As a result, it is critical in the anti-aging process to understand whether you get adequate sleep to allow your body to do what it needs to do to preserve not only your health but also the condition of your skin.

Do You Have Enough Sleep?
Doctors will tell you that you need at least eight hours of sleep each night. Because everyone is different, your body may need more or less. It's easy to tell if you're getting sufficient. Do you feel refreshed when you wake up in the morning? Or do you wake up tired and wish you can sleep for a few more minutes? Your body cannot function properly if you do not get enough sleep. So, look for ways to improve your sleep.

Effective Tips to Help You Fall Asleep Faster

• Avoid eating food or even high-sugar snacks at least two hours before bedtime because they will spike your blood sugar and keep you awake.

• Play white noise, which can be natural sounds or relaxation recordings. Meditation before bedtime is extremely beneficial.

• Avoid watching movies before going to bed. Television stimulates the mind, keeping it alert and thinking. Find a comfortable activity to do instead.

A good night's rest is essential for people who are using anti-aging techniques or who simply want to enhance their general well-being. Learn what it can do for you by going to bed earlier and getting the sleep your body needs. It can also be an excellent complement to other anti-aging techniques.

Chapter 25

Considerations for Anti-Aging Cosmetic Surgery

Take into account who you are looking for if you are considering cosmetic surgery for the finest anti-aging solutions for your needs. When it comes to fixing your body's effects of aging, there are many things to keep in mind. Even though cosmetic surgery may be the perfect idea for you, you should also understand the feelings side of the equation. There may be more to your requirements than cosmetic surgery.

Is Cosmetic Surgery a Good Deal?

There are numerous cosmetic surgeries available to help you continue improving your body's health and appearance.

From a cosmetic standpoint, there is little speculation that a few of these surgeries can improve your health. But, before you can do so, you must first take the time to consider why you want to boost. You should also consider why you want to get this surgery in the first place. Cosmetic surgery may be needed for some people to be happy about themselves. You may only want to slow the effects of aging, such as crow's feet.

However, for others, the process is carried out due to a lack of self-esteem, which can be detrimental in the long run if not handled. What is your position? Are you looking for a few touch-ups to make you look younger, or are you dealing with aging? Do you struggle with self-esteem?

There are numerous compelling reasons to invest in cosmetic surgery. It can be a fantastic way to regain some of the lost self-esteem. Those who continue to improve or who desire a fantastic body and will go to incredible lengths to obtain it are often unconfident and, in some cases, depressed.

In these situations, it is critical to assess why this is the case and then strive to improve it. Cosmetic surgery is an excellent anti-aging treatment.

However, it is not the only tool available to you. Those who do experience other psychological issues will be able to feel and look younger if they seek help and treatment. Indeed, those who are psychologically healthy are often able to overcome health challenges and enhance their overall physical and mental well-being.

Conclusion

Finally, humanity has been on a never-ending hunt for anti-aging, wrinkle, and skincare solutions throughout history. With advances in science, technology, and medicine, we now have a better understanding of the causes of aging and how to halt the process and improve the appearance of our skin. We've learned along the way that the key to youthful skin rests not just in external treatments, but also in internal variables like nutrition, exercise, stress management, and enough sleep. We've discovered that a thorough skincare regimen includes a healthy lifestyle, a consistent skincare routine, and the use of effective anti-aging products. As we become older, it's vital to accept the changes that come with the territory while still taking care of our skin and bodies. We may keep our young glow and enjoy the benefits of healthy, bright skin for years to come by prioritizing self-care and taking a holistic approach to aging. Finally, the most effective anti-aging remedy is a dedication to taking care of ourselves from the inside out, rather than a miracle product or a quick fix. We may mature gracefully and boldly by investing in our health and well-being, understanding that our beauty comes from within.

www.ingramcontent.com/pod-product-compliance
Lightning Source LLC
Chambersburg PA
CBHW070839250726
48662CB00003B/1290